AMELIA WESTWOOD

Pregnancy Myths and Facts

Separating Truth from Tradition for a Healthy Pregnancy Journey"

Contents

Introduction

Understanding Pregnancy Myths and Facts

Introduction

Pregnancy is a time of immense joy and transformation, but it is also a period fraught with uncertainty. Expecting mothers are often bombarded with a plethora of information, some of which is based on myths and misconceptions rather than scientific evidence. This document aims to unravel the truth behind common pregnancy myths, providing clear, evidence-based facts to help guide expectant mothers through this crucial time. By understanding and addressing these myths, we can ensure that pregnant women receive the best possible care and support.

Common Pregnancy Myths

Myth 1: "You're Eating for Two"
One of the most pervasive myths about pregnancy is that a woman should eat for two. This saying suggests that pregnant women need to consume double the amount of food to nourish

both themselves and their baby.

Fact: While it's true that a pregnant woman's caloric needs increase, the actual increase is modest. The American College of Obstetricians and Gynecologists (ACOG) recommends an additional 300–500 calories per day during the second and third trimesters. The focus should be on the quality of food rather than quantity. Nutrient-dense foods rich in vitamins, minerals, and proteins are essential for a healthy pregnancy. Excessive weight gain can lead to complications such as gestational diabetes and hypertension.

Myth 2: "Cravings Predict Baby's Gender"

Many people believe that a mother's food cravings can indicate the sex of her baby. For instance, cravings for sweet foods are often thought to suggest a girl, while cravings for salty or sour foods are believed to indicate a boy.

Fact: There is no scientific evidence to support the idea that cravings can predict a baby's gender. Cravings during pregnancy are more likely influenced by hormonal changes, nutritional deficiencies, and the body's increased energy needs. Gender prediction is best left to medical methods like ultrasound and genetic testing.

Myth 3: "Exercise is Dangerous During Pregnancy"

A common myth is that physical activity can harm the baby or lead to complications. This belief might stem from concerns about physical strain and the risk of injury.

Fact: Exercise is generally safe and beneficial during pregnancy. The ACOG recommends regular, moderate exercise for most pregnant women, unless contraindicated by medical conditions. Exercise can improve overall health, reduce pregnancy-related discomfort, enhance mood, and help manage weight. It's important for expecting mothers to consult with their healthcare provider to tailor an exercise plan that suits their individual needs and conditions.

Myth 4: "Heartburn Means Your Baby Will Have Lots of Hair"

An old wives' tale suggests that severe heartburn during pregnancy is a sign that the baby will be born with a lot of hair.

Fact: There is no scientific correlation between heartburn and the amount of hair a baby will have. Heartburn occurs due to hormonal changes and the physical pressure of the growing uterus on the stomach. It can be managed with dietary changes and medications prescribed by a healthcare provider. The amount of hair a baby has is determined by genetics, not maternal heartburn.

Myth 5: "You Can't Fly While Pregnant"

Some believe that flying during pregnancy is risky and should be avoided altogether.

Fact: Air travel is generally safe for pregnant women, especially during the second trimester. Most airlines have policies accommodating pregnant travelers, but it's important to check with your airline and healthcare provider before flying. Certain medical conditions or complications might necessitate avoiding air travel. Adequate hydration, movement, and proper medical advice can help ensure a safe flight.

Myth-Busting: The Facts Behind Common Misconceptions

Fact 1: Nutritional Needs During Pregnancy

Pregnancy does increase caloric needs, but the additional calories required are modest. Nutritional needs focus on the intake of specific nutrients such as folic acid, iron, calcium, and protein, rather than merely increasing calorie consumption. Balanced meals with a variety of fruits, vegetables, whole grains, lean proteins, and healthy fats can provide the necessary nutrients for both mother and baby.

Fact 2: Cravings and Gender Prediction

Cravings are a normal part of pregnancy and often reflect changes in the body's nutritional requirements. They are not linked to the baby's gender. Gender prediction through non-scientific means lacks evidence and is not reliable. Ultrasound and genetic testing remain the most accurate methods for determining a baby's sex.

Fact 3: Safe Exercise During Pregnancy

Regular exercise, such as walking, swimming, and prenatal yoga, can be beneficial during pregnancy. It helps in managing weight, improving mood, and preparing the body for labor. Pregnant women should avoid high-risk activities and consult their healthcare provider to adapt their exercise routine to their specific situation.

Fact 4: Heartburn and Hair Growth

Heartburn is a common symptom during pregnancy due to hormonal and physical changes. It is not an indicator of the baby's hair quantity. Managing heartburn involves dietary adjustments and medical advice rather than relying on old wives' tales.

Fact 5: Air Travel and Pregnancy Safety

Air travel is safe for most pregnant women, especially in the second trimester. Pregnant women should follow general travel guidelines, such as staying hydrated and moving around during long flights. Consulting with a healthcare provider before flying is recommended to address any personal health concerns.

Cultural and Historical Perspectives on Pregnancy Myths

Ancient Beliefs and Practices

Throughout history, pregnancy has been surrounded by various beliefs and practices. In ancient cultures, myths and rituals were often used to explain and influence pregnancy and childbirth. For example, some cultures believed that specific foods or actions could affect the baby's health or gender.

Modern Cultural Influences

Modern cultural influences continue to perpetuate pregnancy myths through media, social traditions, and family beliefs. The spread of misinformation can impact pregnant women's decisions and health. It's essential to differentiate between cultural traditions and evidence-based medical advice.

Impact on Expecting Mothers Across Cultures

Cultural beliefs about pregnancy can vary widely and affect how expecting mothers approach prenatal care. Understanding these cultural perspectives can help healthcare providers offer more personalized and respectful care, addressing both medical needs and cultural sensitivities.

The Science Behind Pregnancy Facts

The Role of Nutrition and Dietary Guidelines

Scientific research emphasizes the importance of a balanced diet during pregnancy. Essential nutrients such as folic acid, iron, calcium, and omega-3 fatty acids support fetal development and maternal health. Guidelines provided by organizations like the Dietary Guidelines for Americans and the World Health Organization outline the necessary nutritional adjustments for a healthy pregnancy.

Exercise Recommendations and Research

Research supports the benefits of regular exercise during pregnancy. Studies have shown that moderate physical activity can reduce the risk of gestational diabetes, improve mood, and facilitate labor. Exercise guidelines provided by the ACOG and other health organizations recommend incorporating activities that are safe and enjoyable for pregnant women.

Hormonal Changes and Physical Symptoms

Pregnancy induces significant hormonal changes that affect various bodily functions. Understanding these changes helps in managing common symptoms such as nausea, fatigue, and heartburn. Research into hormonal impacts provides insight into managing these symptoms and ensuring a healthier pregnancy experience.

Expert Opinions and Medical Advice

Interviews with Obstetricians and Gynecologists

Healthcare professionals, including obstetricians and gynecologists, provide valuable insights into pregnancy management. Interviews with experts can clarify misconceptions, offer practical advice, and address common concerns about pregnancy myths.

Insights from Nutritionists and Fitness Experts

Nutritionists and fitness experts offer guidance on maintaining a balanced diet and safe exercise routines during pregnancy. Their expertise helps in understanding the importance of proper nutrition and physical activity in supporting a healthy pregnancy.

Real-Life Experiences from Expecting Mothers

Personal stories from expecting mothers can provide relatable insights into managing pregnancy. These experiences highlight the real-world impact of myths and facts, offering practical advice and emotional support.

Practical Tips for Navigating Pregnancy Information

How to Distinguish Between Fact and Fiction

Navigating pregnancy information requires critical thinking and skepticism. Checking sources, consulting healthcare providers, and relying on evidence-based information can help in distinguishing between accurate facts and myths.

Reliable Sources for Pregnancy Information

Reliable sources include medical journals, official health organization guidelines, and reputable healthcare providers. Avoiding unverified online sources and consulting with professionals ensures access to accurate and up-to-date information.

Addressing Concerns with Your Healthcare Provider

Open communication with healthcare providers is crucial for addressing concerns and clarifying doubts. Discussing any myths or misconceptions with a healthcare professional ensures that pregnant women receive evidence-based advice tailored to their individual needs.

Case Studies and Personal Stories

Experiences of Women Who Debunked Myths

Personal stories of women who have navigated pregnancy myths can provide valuable lessons and encouragement. These case studies highlight the importance of seeking accurate information and making informed decisions.

Lessons Learned from Personal Journeys

Reflecting on personal experiences helps in understanding the impact of myths and facts on pregnancy. Lessons learned can offer guidance and reassurance to other expecting mothers.

Resources for Further Reading

Recommended Books and Articles

Books and articles from reputable sources provide in-depth information on pregnancy myths and facts. Recommendations can include texts by experts in obstetrics, nutrition, and maternal health.

Online Resources and Support Groups

Online resources and support groups offer additional information and community support for expecting mothers. Websites, forums, and social media groups can provide valuable advice and shared experiences.

Educational Websites and Apps

Educational websites and apps designed for pregnancy provide interactive tools and information. These resources can help in tracking pregnancy progress, accessing reliable information, and connecting with other expectant mothers.

Conclusion

Embracing Accurate Information for a Healthy Pregnancy

Understanding and addressing pregnancy myths is essential for ensuring a healthy and informed pregnancy. Embracing accurate, evidence-based information helps expectant mothers make better decisions and receive appropriate care.

Moving Beyond Myths for Better Prenatal Care

By moving beyond myths and focusing on facts, pregnant

women can improve their prenatal care experience. Collaborating with healthcare providers, seeking reliable information, and staying informed will contribute to a healthier pregnancy and better outcomes for both mother and baby.

The Importance of Accurate Information in Pregnancy

Introduction

Pregnancy is a transformative period in a woman's life, filled with anticipation, joy, and a myriad of questions and concerns. Amid the excitement, expectant mothers are often bombarded with information—some of it accurate, some of it misleading or incorrect. The significance of accurate information during pregnancy cannot be overstated. Accurate information ensures that expectant mothers make informed decisions about their health, their baby's health, and their overall pregnancy experience. This comprehensive exploration will delve into why accurate information is crucial, how misinformation can impact pregnancy, and how to access reliable resources.

The Impact of Accurate Information

1. Informed Decision-Making

Accurate information empowers expectant mothers to make informed decisions regarding their prenatal care, nutrition, and lifestyle. Knowledge about the following areas is crucial:

- **Prenatal Care:** Understanding what to expect during prenatal visits, the importance of routine screenings, and when to seek medical advice helps in ensuring both maternal and fetal health. Accurate information on prenatal vitamins, screening tests, and vaccinations is vital for a healthy pregnancy.
- **Nutrition:** Proper nutrition is fundamental to a healthy pregnancy. Accurate information about nutritional needs, safe foods, and dietary restrictions helps prevent complications such as gestational diabetes and nutritional deficiencies.
- **Labor and Delivery:** Knowing what to expect during labor and delivery, including pain management options and potential complications, prepares expectant mothers for the birthing process and helps in making choices about their birth plan.

2. Managing Health and Safety

Accurate information is essential for managing health and safety throughout pregnancy. It helps in:

- **Avoiding Risks:** Understanding potential risks and warning signs of complications, such as preeclampsia or preterm labor, allows for timely intervention and reduces the risk of adverse outcomes.
- **Medication and Treatment:** Accurate information about the safety and effects of medications and treatments during pregnancy is crucial. It ensures that expectant mothers make safe choices regarding over-the-counter and prescription medications.
- **Mental Health:** Pregnancy can bring about emotional and

psychological changes. Accurate information on mental health resources and coping strategies helps in managing stress, anxiety, and depression, contributing to overall well-being.

The Dangers of Misinformation

1. Misguided Decisions

Misinformation can lead to misguided decisions that may negatively impact pregnancy and fetal health:

- **Nutritional Myths:** Believing in myths about dietary restrictions or excessive caloric intake can lead to poor nutritional choices, potentially resulting in complications such as gestational diabetes or inadequate fetal growth.
- **Exercise Misconceptions:** Misunderstanding exercise guidelines can lead to either excessive or insufficient physical activity, impacting maternal fitness and overall health. Accurate information helps in maintaining a balanced and safe exercise routine.
- **Medical Procedures:** Incorrect information about medical procedures, such as ultrasounds or labor induction, can lead to unnecessary anxiety or reluctance to pursue necessary treatments. Understanding the purpose and safety of these procedures is crucial for informed decision-making.

2. Health Risks

Misinformation poses health risks for both the mother and the baby:

- **Complications:** Believing in myths or outdated practices can increase the risk of complications. For example, avoiding certain foods due to incorrect beliefs may lead to nutrient deficiencies or foodborne illnesses.

- **Preventative Measures:** Misinformation can lead to neglect of essential preventive measures, such as vaccinations or screenings, increasing the risk of preventable health issues.
- **Mental Health:** Misinformation about mental health during pregnancy can exacerbate stress and anxiety, affecting overall well-being and potentially leading to conditions such as prenatal or postpartum depression.

Accessing Reliable Information

1. Consult Healthcare Professionals

Healthcare professionals, including obstetricians, gynecologists, and midwives, are primary sources of reliable information. They provide evidence-based guidance tailored to individual needs. Engaging in open communication with healthcare providers ensures that concerns are addressed and accurate advice is given.

- **Regular Check-Ups:** Routine prenatal visits offer opportunities to discuss any questions or concerns with a healthcare provider. These visits also provide a chance to receive personalized advice and guidance.
- **Specialist Referrals:** In cases of complex or high-risk pregnancies, referrals to specialists such as maternal-fetal medicine experts or nutritionists can provide additional insights and support.

2. Utilize Reputable Resources

Reliable information can also be obtained from reputable resources, including:

- **Medical Websites:** Websites of organizations such as the American College of Obstetricians and Gynecologists (ACOG), the Centers for Disease Control and Prevention (CDC), and the World Health Organization (WHO) offer evidence-based information on pregnancy-related topics.
- **Educational Materials:** Books and articles authored by experts in obstetrics, nutrition, and prenatal care provide valuable information. Ensure that these materials are up-to-date and authored by credible professionals.
- **Support Groups:** Online and in-person support groups for expecting mothers can provide community support and share experiences. While these can be valuable, it's essential to cross-reference information with reliable sources.

3. Avoid Misinformation
To avoid misinformation:

- **Verify Sources:** Check the credibility of sources before accepting information. Avoid relying on anecdotal evidence or unverified online posts.
- **Consult Professionals:** When in doubt, consult healthcare professionals to clarify any conflicting information or address specific concerns.
- **Be Skeptical:** Approach information with a critical mindset, especially if it seems too good to be true or contradicts established medical guidelines.

The Role of Education and Awareness

1. Promoting Health Literacy
   Health literacy is crucial for understanding and using health information effectively. Promoting health literacy among expectant mothers helps in:

- **Empowering Women:** Educating women about pregnancy, prenatal care, and childbirth empowers them to make informed decisions and actively participate in their care.
- **Improving Outcomes:** Enhanced health literacy is associated with better pregnancy outcomes, as informed women are more likely to engage in healthy behaviors and seek timely medical care.
- **Reducing Misconceptions:** Education helps in debunking myths and misconceptions, leading to better adherence to evidence-based practices.

2. Public Health Campaigns
   Public health campaigns play a vital role in disseminating accurate information:

- **Educational Programs:** Programs aimed at educating pregnant women about nutrition, exercise, and prenatal care can improve health outcomes and reduce the spread of misinformation.
- **Media Campaigns:** Media campaigns that provide accurate and accessible information can reach a broad audience, helping to address common myths and promote evidence-based practices.
- **Community Outreach:**   Engaging with communities

through workshops, seminars, and support groups can facilitate the dissemination of accurate information and foster a supportive environment for expectant mothers.

Conclusion

The importance of accurate information during pregnancy cannot be overstated. Accurate information empowers expectant mothers to make informed decisions, manage health and safety effectively, and avoid the pitfalls of misinformation. By consulting healthcare professionals, utilizing reputable resources, and promoting health literacy, expectant mothers can navigate their pregnancy with confidence and ensure the best possible outcomes for themselves and their babies.

In a world where information is abundant but not always reliable, the responsibility falls on both healthcare providers and expectant mothers to seek out and uphold accurate, evidence-based information. Embracing this approach not only enhances the pregnancy experience but also supports a healthier and happier journey into motherhood.The Importance of Accurate Information in Pregnancy

Introduction

Pregnancy is a transformative period in a woman's life, filled with anticipation, joy, and a myriad of questions and concerns. Amid the excitement, expectant mothers are often bombarded with information—some of it accurate, some of it misleading or incorrect. The significance of accurate information during pregnancy cannot be overstated. Accurate information ensures that expectant mothers make informed decisions about their health, their baby's health, and their overall pregnancy experience. This comprehensive exploration will delve into why accurate information is crucial, how misinformation can impact pregnancy, and how to access reliable resources.

The Impact of Accurate Information

1. Informed Decision-Making

Accurate information empowers expectant mothers to make informed decisions regarding their prenatal care, nutrition, and lifestyle. Knowledge about the following areas is crucial:

· **Prenatal Care:** Understanding what to expect during prenatal visits, the importance of routine screenings, and when to seek medical advice helps in ensuring both maternal and fetal health. Accurate information on prenatal vitamins, screening tests, and vaccinations is vital for a healthy pregnancy.

- **Nutrition:** Proper nutrition is fundamental to a healthy pregnancy. Accurate information about nutritional needs, safe foods, and dietary restrictions helps prevent complications such as gestational diabetes and nutritional deficiencies.
- **Labor and Delivery:** Knowing what to expect during labor and delivery, including pain management options and potential complications, prepares expectant mothers for the birthing process and helps in making choices about their birth plan.

2. Managing Health and Safety

Accurate information is essential for managing health and safety throughout pregnancy. It helps in:

- **Avoiding Risks:** Understanding potential risks and warning signs of complications, such as preeclampsia or preterm labor, allows for timely intervention and reduces the risk of adverse outcomes.
- **Medication and Treatment:** Accurate information about the safety and effects of medications and treatments during pregnancy is crucial. It ensures that expectant mothers make safe choices regarding over-the-counter and prescription medications.
- **Mental Health:** Pregnancy can bring about emotional and psychological changes. Accurate information on mental

health resources and coping strategies helps in managing stress, anxiety, and depression, contributing to overall well-being.

The Dangers of Misinformation

1. Misguided Decisions

Misinformation can lead to misguided decisions that may negatively impact pregnancy and fetal health:

- **Nutritional Myths:** Believing in myths about dietary restrictions or excessive caloric intake can lead to poor nutritional choices, potentially resulting in complications such as gestational diabetes or inadequate fetal growth.
- **Exercise Misconceptions:** Misunderstanding exercise guidelines can lead to either excessive or insufficient physical activity, impacting maternal fitness and overall health. Accurate information helps in maintaining a balanced and safe exercise routine.
- **Medical Procedures:** Incorrect information about medical procedures, such as ultrasounds or labor induction, can lead to unnecessary anxiety or reluctance to pursue necessary treatments. Understanding the purpose and safety of these procedures is crucial for informed decision-making.

2. Health Risks

Misinformation poses health risks for both the mother and the baby:

- **Complications:** Believing in myths or outdated practices can increase the risk of complications. For example, avoiding certain foods due to incorrect beliefs may lead to nutrient deficiencies or foodborne illnesses.

- **Preventative Measures:** Misinformation can lead to neglect of essential preventive measures, such as vaccinations or screenings, increasing the risk of preventable health issues.
- **Mental Health:** Misinformation about mental health during pregnancy can exacerbate stress and anxiety, affecting overall well-being and potentially leading to conditions such as prenatal or postpartum depression.

Accessing Reliable Information

1. Consult Healthcare Professionals

Healthcare professionals, including obstetricians, gynecologists, and midwives, are primary sources of reliable information. They provide evidence-based guidance tailored to individual needs. Engaging in open communication with healthcare providers ensures that concerns are addressed and accurate advice is given.

- **Regular Check-Ups:** Routine prenatal visits offer opportunities to discuss any questions or concerns with a healthcare provider. These visits also provide a chance to receive personalized advice and guidance.
- **Specialist Referrals:** In cases of complex or high-risk pregnancies, referrals to specialists such as maternal-fetal medicine experts or nutritionists can provide additional insights and support.

2. Utilize Reputable Resources

Reliable information can also be obtained from reputable

resources, including:

- **Medical Websites:** Websites of organizations such as the American College of Obstetricians and Gynecologists (ACOG), the Centers for Disease Control and Prevention (CDC), and the World Health Organization (WHO) offer evidence-based information on pregnancy-related topics.
- **Educational Materials:** Books and articles authored by experts in obstetrics, nutrition, and prenatal care provide valuable information. Ensure that these materials are up-to-date and authored by credible professionals.
- **Support Groups:** Online and in-person support groups for expecting mothers can provide community support and share experiences. While these can be valuable, it's essential to cross-reference information with reliable sources.

3. Avoid Misinformation

To avoid misinformation:

- **Verify Sources:** Check the credibility of sources before accepting information. Avoid relying on anecdotal evidence or unverified online posts.
- **Consult Professionals:** When in doubt, consult healthcare professionals to clarify any conflicting information or address specific concerns.
- **Be Skeptical:** Approach information with a critical mindset, especially if it seems too good to be true or contradicts established medical guidelines.

The Role of Education and Awareness

1. Promoting Health Literacy

Health literacy is crucial for understanding and using health information effectively. Promoting health literacy among expectant mothers helps in:

- **Empowering Women:** Educating women about pregnancy, prenatal care, and childbirth empowers them to make informed decisions and actively participate in their care.
- **Improving Outcomes:** Enhanced health literacy is associated with better pregnancy outcomes, as informed women are more likely to engage in healthy behaviors and seek timely medical care.
- **Reducing Misconceptions:** Education helps in debunking myths and misconceptions, leading to better adherence to evidence-based practices.

2. Public Health Campaigns

Public health campaigns play a vital role in disseminating accurate information:

- **Educational Programs:** Programs aimed at educating pregnant women about nutrition, exercise, and prenatal care can improve health outcomes and reduce the spread of misinformation.
- **Media Campaigns:** Media campaigns that provide accurate and accessible information can reach a broad audience, helping to address common myths and promote evidence-based practices.
- **Community Outreach:** Engaging with communities

through workshops, seminars, and support groups can facilitate the dissemination of accurate information and foster a supportive environment for expectant mothers.

Conclusion

The importance of accurate information during pregnancy cannot be overstated. Accurate information empowers expectant mothers to make informed decisions, manage health and safety effectively, and avoid the pitfalls of misinformation. By consulting healthcare professionals, utilizing reputable resources, and promoting health literacy, expectant mothers can navigate their pregnancy with confidence and ensure the best possible outcomes for themselves and their babies.

In a world where information is abundant but not always reliable, the responsibility falls on both healthcare providers and expectant mothers to seek out and uphold accurate, evidence-based information. Embracing this approach not only enhances the pregnancy experience but also supports a healthier and happier journey into motherhood.The Importance of Accurate Information in Pregnancy

Introduction

Pregnancy is a transformative period in a woman's life, filled with anticipation, joy, and a myriad of questions and concerns. Amid the excitement, expectant mothers are often bombarded with information—some of it accurate, some of it misleading or incorrect. The significance of accurate information during pregnancy cannot be overstated. Accurate information ensures that expectant mothers make informed decisions about their health, their baby's health, and their overall pregnancy experience. This comprehensive exploration will delve into why accurate information is crucial, how misinformation can impact pregnancy, and how to access reliable resources.

The Impact of Accurate Information

1. Informed Decision-Making

Accurate information empowers expectant mothers to make informed decisions regarding their prenatal care, nutrition, and lifestyle. Knowledge about the following areas is crucial:

- **Prenatal Care:** Understanding what to expect during prenatal visits, the importance of routine screenings, and when to seek medical advice helps in ensuring both maternal and fetal health. Accurate information on prenatal vitamins, screening tests, and vaccinations is vital for a healthy pregnancy.

- **Nutrition:** Proper nutrition is fundamental to a healthy pregnancy. Accurate information about nutritional needs, safe foods, and dietary restrictions helps prevent complications such as gestational diabetes and nutritional deficiencies.

- **Labor and Delivery:** Knowing what to expect during labor and delivery, including pain management options and potential complications, prepares expectant mothers for the birthing process and helps in making choices about their birth plan.

2. Managing Health and Safety

Accurate information is essential for managing health and safety throughout pregnancy. It helps in:

- **Avoiding Risks:** Understanding potential risks and warning signs of complications, such as preeclampsia or preterm labor, allows for timely intervention and reduces the risk of adverse outcomes.

- **Medication and Treatment:** Accurate information about the safety and effects of medications and treatments during pregnancy is crucial. It ensures that expectant mothers make safe choices regarding over-the-counter and prescription medications.

- **Mental Health:** Pregnancy can bring about emotional and psychological changes. Accurate information on mental health resources and coping strategies helps in managing stress, anxiety, and depression, contributing to overall well-being.

The Dangers of Misinformation

1. Misguided Decisions

Misinformation can lead to misguided decisions that may negatively impact pregnancy and fetal health:

- **Nutritional Myths:** Believing in myths about dietary restrictions or excessive caloric intake can lead to poor nutritional choices, potentially resulting in complications such as gestational diabetes or inadequate fetal growth.
- **Exercise Misconceptions:** Misunderstanding exercise guidelines can lead to either excessive or insufficient physical activity, impacting maternal fitness and overall health. Accurate information helps in maintaining a balanced and safe exercise routine.
- **Medical Procedures:** Incorrect information about medical procedures, such as ultrasounds or labor induction, can lead to unnecessary anxiety or reluctance to pursue necessary treatments. Understanding the purpose and safety of these procedures is crucial for informed decision-making.

2. Health Risks

Misinformation poses health risks for both the mother and the baby:

- **Complications:** Believing in myths or outdated practices can increase the risk of complications. For example, avoiding certain foods due to incorrect beliefs may lead to nutrient deficiencies or foodborne illnesses.

- **Preventative Measures:** Misinformation can lead to neglect of essential preventive measures, such as vaccinations or screenings, increasing the risk of preventable health issues.
- **Mental Health:** Misinformation about mental health during pregnancy can exacerbate stress and anxiety, affecting overall well-being and potentially leading to conditions such as prenatal or postpartum depression.

Accessing Reliable Information

1. Consult Healthcare Professionals

Healthcare professionals, including obstetricians, gynecologists, and midwives, are primary sources of reliable information. They provide evidence-based guidance tailored to individual needs. Engaging in open communication with healthcare providers ensures that concerns are addressed and accurate advice is given.

- **Regular Check-Ups:** Routine prenatal visits offer opportunities to discuss any questions or concerns with a healthcare provider. These visits also provide a chance to receive personalized advice and guidance.
- **Specialist Referrals:** In cases of complex or high-risk pregnancies, referrals to specialists such as maternal-fetal medicine experts or nutritionists can provide additional insights and support.

2. Utilize Reputable Resources

Reliable information can also be obtained from reputable

resources, including:

- **Medical Websites:** Websites of organizations such as the American College of Obstetricians and Gynecologists (ACOG), the Centers for Disease Control and Prevention (CDC), and the World Health Organization (WHO) offer evidence-based information on pregnancy-related topics.
- **Educational Materials:** Books and articles authored by experts in obstetrics, nutrition, and prenatal care provide valuable information. Ensure that these materials are up-to-date and authored by credible professionals.
- **Support Groups:** Online and in-person support groups for expecting mothers can provide community support and share experiences. While these can be valuable, it's essential to cross-reference information with reliable sources.

3. Avoid Misinformation
   To avoid misinformation:

- **Verify Sources:** Check the credibility of sources before accepting information. Avoid relying on anecdotal evidence or unverified online posts.
- **Consult Professionals:** When in doubt, consult healthcare professionals to clarify any conflicting information or address specific concerns.
- **Be Skeptical:** Approach information with a critical mindset, especially if it seems too good to be true or contradicts established medical guidelines.

The Role of Education and Awareness

1. Promoting Health Literacy

Health literacy is crucial for understanding and using health information effectively. Promoting health literacy among expectant mothers helps in:

- **Empowering Women:** Educating women about pregnancy, prenatal care, and childbirth empowers them to make informed decisions and actively participate in their care.
- **Improving Outcomes:** Enhanced health literacy is associated with better pregnancy outcomes, as informed women are more likely to engage in healthy behaviors and seek timely medical care.
- **Reducing Misconceptions:** Education helps in debunking myths and misconceptions, leading to better adherence to evidence-based practices.

2. Public Health Campaigns

Public health campaigns play a vital role in disseminating accurate information:

- **Educational Programs:** Programs aimed at educating pregnant women about nutrition, exercise, and prenatal care can improve health outcomes and reduce the spread of misinformation.
- **Media Campaigns:** Media campaigns that provide accurate and accessible information can reach a broad audience, helping to address common myths and promote evidence-based practices.
- **Community Outreach:** Engaging with communities

through workshops, seminars, and support groups can facilitate the dissemination of accurate information and foster a supportive environment for expectant mothers.

Conclusion

The importance of accurate information during pregnancy cannot be overstated. Accurate information empowers expectant mothers to make informed decisions, manage health and safety effectively, and avoid the pitfalls of misinformation. By consulting healthcare professionals, utilizing reputable resources, and promoting health literacy, expectant mothers can navigate their pregnancy with confidence and ensure the best possible outcomes for themselves and their babies.

In a world where information is abundant but not always reliable, the responsibility falls on both healthcare providers and expectant mothers to seek out and uphold accurate, evidence-based information. Embracing this approach not only enhances the pregnancy experience but also supports a healthier and happier journey into motherhood.

Common Pregnancy Myths

Myth 1: "You're Eating for Two"

Introduction

One of the most pervasive and misleading myths about pregnancy is the idea that a woman needs to "eat for two." This concept implies that pregnant women should double their food intake to meet the needs of both themselves and their developing baby. This myth is not only inaccurate but can also lead to unhealthy eating habits and complications. In this detailed examination, we will explore the origins of this myth, the actual nutritional needs during pregnancy, and the potential impacts of misunderstanding this concept.

Origins of the Myth

The idea that pregnant women should eat for two has been around for centuries and is rooted in cultural beliefs and outdated practices. Historically, pregnancy was often viewed as a period where a woman needed to consume extra food to ensure both her health and the health of her baby. This belief was partly due to limited understanding of nutritional science and a lack of emphasis on balanced diets.

In the early 20th century, this notion gained further traction through popular culture and media, which often portrayed pregnancy as a time for indulgence and increased caloric intake. The phrase "eating for two" became a common mantra, reinforcing the idea that expectant mothers needed to consume significantly more food.

Nutritional Needs During Pregnancy

Increased Caloric Intake

While it is true that a woman's caloric needs increase during pregnancy, the amount is often less than what the myth suggests. According to the American College of Obstetricians and Gynecologists (ACOG), the additional caloric intake recommended during pregnancy is approximately 300-500 calories per day, particularly during the second and third trimesters. This increase is intended to support the energy needs of the growing fetus and the physiological changes occurring in the mother's body.

However, this increase does not mean doubling food intake. The focus should be on the quality of calories consumed rather than simply increasing quantity. Nutrient-dense foods that provide essential vitamins, minerals, and other nutrients are crucial for a healthy pregnancy.

Essential Nutrients

Pregnant women require a range of essential nutrients to support fetal development and maternal health. Key nutrients include:

- **Folic Acid:** Vital for preventing neural tube defects and supporting fetal growth. Recommended intake is 400-800 micrograms per day.
- **Iron:** Necessary for the increased blood volume and to prevent anemia. The recommended intake is 27 milligrams per day.
- **Calcium:** Supports the development of the baby's bones and teeth. The recommended intake is 1,000 milligrams per day.
- **Protein:** Important for the growth of fetal tissues, including the brain. The recommended intake is about 71 grams per day.
- **Omega-3 Fatty Acids:** Supports brain development and reduces the risk of preterm birth. Sources include fatty fish and supplements.

A balanced diet that includes fruits, vegetables, whole grains, lean proteins, and healthy fats can help meet these nutritional needs.

Risks of Overeating

Excessive Weight Gain
The myth of "eating for two" can lead to excessive weight gain, which is associated with several risks, including:

- **Gestational Diabetes:** Overeating can contribute to the development of gestational diabetes, a condition characterized by high blood sugar levels during pregnancy.
- **Hypertension:** Excessive weight gain increases the risk of developing pregnancy-related hypertension, which can lead to complications such as preeclampsia.

- **Difficulty During Labor:** Excessive weight gain can complicate labor and delivery, increasing the likelihood of a cesarean section.

Maintaining a healthy weight gain is important for reducing these risks and ensuring a healthy pregnancy. The recommended weight gain varies based on pre-pregnancy body mass index (BMI) and other individual factors.

Nutritional Imbalance

Focusing on quantity rather than quality of food can lead to nutritional imbalances. For example, consuming large amounts of high-calorie, low-nutrient foods can result in deficiencies in essential vitamins and minerals. This can impact both maternal health and fetal development.

Healthy Eating Guidelines

Focus on Nutrient-Dense Foods

To meet increased nutritional needs during pregnancy, it is essential to prioritize nutrient-dense foods:

- **Fruits and Vegetables:** Provide essential vitamins, minerals, and fiber. Aim for a variety of colors to ensure a broad range of nutrients.
- **Whole Grains:** Offer fiber, B vitamins, and minerals. Choose whole grains over refined grains for better nutritional value.
- **Lean Proteins:** Support fetal growth and repair tissues. Sources include poultry, fish, beans, and tofu.
- **Dairy Products:** Provide calcium and protein. Opt for low-fat or fat-free options to reduce saturated fat intake.

Portion Control and Balanced Meals

Managing portion sizes and eating balanced meals helps in meeting nutritional needs without excessive caloric intake:

- **Meal Planning:** Plan meals to include a variety of food groups and ensure balanced nutrient intake.
- **Snacking Wisely:** Choose healthy snacks, such as nuts, yogurt, or fruit, to satisfy hunger and provide additional nutrients.

Hydration and Supplements

Maintaining proper hydration and using prenatal supplements as recommended by a healthcare provider is also important:

- **Hydration:** Drinking adequate water supports overall health and helps in managing pregnancy symptoms such as swelling.
- **Prenatal Vitamins:** Taking prenatal vitamins ensures adequate intake of essential nutrients, especially if dietary intake is insufficient.

Addressing the Myth

Educating Expectant Mothers

Education plays a key role in dispelling the myth of "eating for two." Healthcare providers can offer guidance on:

- **Caloric Needs:** Clarifying the modest increase in caloric intake and emphasizing the importance of nutrient quality.
- **Healthy Eating Habits:** Providing practical advice on meal

planning, portion control, and choosing nutrient-dense foods.

Promoting Evidence-Based Practices
Promoting evidence-based practices helps in aligning dietary recommendations with scientific research:

- **Guidelines and Resources:** Utilizing guidelines from reputable organizations, such as the ACOG and the Academy of Nutrition and Dietetics, to provide accurate information.
- **Support and Counseling:** Offering nutritional counseling and support to address individual needs and concerns.

Conclusion

The myth of "eating for two" can lead to misconceptions about pregnancy nutrition and result in unhealthy eating habits and potential complications. Accurate information about the modest increase in caloric needs, the importance of nutrient-dense foods, and the risks of overeating is essential for a healthy pregnancy. By focusing on balanced meals, portion control, and proper hydration, expectant mothers can meet their nutritional needs and support the health and development of their baby. Education and evidence-based practices are key to dispelling myths and ensuring a healthy and informed pregnancy experience.

Myth 2: "Cravings Predict Baby's Gender"

Introduction

The belief that a mother's food cravings can predict the gender of her baby is a popular myth with deep roots in folklore and cultural traditions. According to this myth, the types of foods a pregnant woman craves—or avoids—are believed to provide clues about whether she is carrying a boy or a girl. This idea is widespread, but it lacks scientific backing. This detailed examination explores the origins of this myth, the scientific perspective on cravings, and how expecting mothers can approach cravings during pregnancy.

Origins of the Myth

Historical and Cultural Beliefs
The notion that food cravings can indicate a baby's gender has been part of folklore in various cultures for centuries. Historically, different cultures have developed their own methods for predicting the sex of an unborn child based on maternal behavior and symptoms. For example:

- **Sweet vs. Salty Cravings:** In some cultures, cravings for sweet foods are thought to signal that the baby is a girl, while cravings for salty or sour foods are believed to indicate a boy. This dichotomy reflects the broader cultural belief that pregnancy cravings are somehow linked to the baby's gender.
- **Traditional Practices:** In other cultures, traditional practices and old wives' tales about gender prediction might

include interpreting maternal cravings along with other symptoms, such as changes in skin complexion or the shape of the mother's belly.

These beliefs often stem from a time when medical knowledge about pregnancy was limited and people relied more on intuition and observation of physical symptoms to understand pregnancy.

The Science Behind Cravings

Hormonal and Physical Changes

Pregnancy induces significant hormonal and physical changes in a woman's body, which can influence her taste preferences and cravings. These changes are not related to the baby's gender but are part of the body's adaptation to pregnancy:

- **Hormones:** Fluctuations in hormones such as progesterone and estrogen can affect taste and smell, leading to changes in food cravings. For example, heightened sensitivity to certain smells and tastes can result in cravings or aversions to specific foods.
- **Nutritional Needs:** Cravings may also be linked to the body's increased nutritional needs during pregnancy. For instance, a craving for certain foods might indicate a need for specific nutrients, such as iron or calcium, rather than an indication of the baby's sex.

Lack of Scientific Evidence

There is no scientific evidence to support the idea that cravings are related to the baby's gender. Research studies on pregnancy cravings have focused on understanding their physiological and psychological aspects rather than linking them to gender prediction. Key points include:

- **Research Findings:** Studies on pregnancy cravings generally focus on their causes, such as hormonal changes, dietary deficiencies, and emotional factors, rather than their correlation with the baby's sex.
- **Expert Opinions:** Healthcare professionals and researchers agree that cravings are a normal part of pregnancy and are not indicative of the baby's gender. Gender determination relies on medical methods such as ultrasounds and genetic testing, which are based on scientific principles.

Understanding and Managing Cravings

Common Cravings During Pregnancy

Cravings during pregnancy are common and can vary widely among women. Some common cravings include:

- **Sweet Foods:** Many pregnant women crave sweet foods, such as chocolate, ice cream, and fruit. This can be attributed to hormonal changes and changes in taste preferences.
- **Salty and Savory Foods:** Cravings for salty or savory foods, like chips or pickles, are also common and can be related to changes in fluid balance and electrolyte needs.
- **Unusual Combinations:** Some women experience cravings for unusual food combinations or non-food items (a condition known as pica). These cravings are often driven by specific nutritional needs or hormonal changes.

Healthy Approaches to Cravings

While cravings themselves are a normal part of pregnancy, managing them healthily is important for maintaining overall well-being:

- **Balanced Diet:** Focus on a balanced diet that includes a variety of nutrients. While it's okay to indulge in cravings occasionally, aim to make healthy choices most of the time.
- **Moderation:** Moderation is key to managing cravings. Satisfy cravings in small amounts and choose healthier alternatives when possible. For example, opt for fruit instead of sugary snacks or whole-grain options instead of refined carbs.
- **Consulting Healthcare Providers:** If cravings are intense or lead to concerns about nutritional deficiencies, consulting with a healthcare provider or a registered dietitian can provide personalized advice and support.

Gender Prediction Methods

Reliable Methods for Determining Gender

Scientific methods for predicting or determining a baby's gender include:

- **Ultrasound:** A common and reliable method for determining the baby's gender is through ultrasound imaging. Typically performed around 18-20 weeks of pregnancy, this method uses sound waves to visualize the baby's anatomy.
- **Genetic Testing:** Tests such as chorionic villus sampling (CVS) and amniocentesis can provide information about the baby's sex by analyzing fetal DNA. These tests are typically

performed for specific medical reasons rather than solely for gender prediction.

- **Non-Invasive Prenatal Testing (NIPT):** NIPT analyzes fetal DNA in the mother's blood to determine the baby's sex with high accuracy. This test can be performed as early as the first trimester.

Myths vs. Facts

Understanding the difference between myths and scientifically supported facts helps in making informed decisions:

- **Myth:** Cravings can predict the baby's gender.
- **Fact:** There is no scientific evidence linking cravings to the baby's sex. Gender prediction relies on medical methods like ultrasounds and genetic testing.

Addressing and Educating About Myths

Educating Expectant Mothers

Education plays a crucial role in dispelling myths about pregnancy:

- **Providing Accurate Information:** Healthcare providers can offer accurate information about pregnancy cravings and gender prediction. Clear explanations help expectant mothers understand the normalcy of cravings and the scientific methods for gender determination.
- **Debunking Myths:** Addressing and debunking myths through education and evidence-based information helps prevent misinformation from affecting pregnancy experiences.

Promoting Evidence-Based Practices

Promoting evidence-based practices ensures that expectant mothers receive reliable information:

- **Medical Guidance:** Rely on medical professionals for accurate information and guidance regarding pregnancy symptoms and gender prediction.
- **Educational Resources:** Utilize reputable sources and educational materials to provide accurate and up-to-date information.

Conclusion

The myth that cravings can predict a baby's gender is a widespread but unfounded belief. Cravings during pregnancy are influenced by hormonal and physical changes rather than the baby's sex. Understanding the scientific basis of cravings, managing them healthily, and relying on reliable methods for gender prediction can help expecting mothers navigate their pregnancy with accurate information. Education and evidence-based practices are essential for dispelling myths and ensuring a well-informed and healthy pregnancy experience.

Myth 3: "Exercise is Dangerous During Pregnancy"

Introduction

The belief that exercise is dangerous during pregnancy is a prevalent myth that has been debunked by modern medical research. Historically, pregnant women were often advised to rest and avoid physical activity to prevent potential complications. However, contemporary understanding of prenatal health emphasizes the numerous benefits of exercise during pregnancy. This comprehensive examination explores the origins of this myth, the current scientific perspective on exercise during pregnancy, and practical guidelines for safe physical activity.

Origins of the Myth

Historical Views on Pregnancy and Exercise

Historically, pregnancy was often associated with the need for rest and limited physical activity. This view was influenced by:

- **Medical Practices:** Early medical practices and beliefs about pregnancy were based on limited scientific knowledge. It was thought that physical activity could harm both the mother and the developing fetus, leading to recommendations for strict bed rest.
- **Cultural Beliefs:** Cultural beliefs and traditions also played a role in shaping attitudes toward exercise during pregnancy. In many cultures, pregnancy was seen as a time to slow down and protect the body from any potential strain.

Shift in Medical Perspective

As medical research advanced, the understanding of pregnancy and exercise began to shift:

- **Emergence of Research:** Research on the benefits of exercise during pregnancy started to emerge, challenging the notion that physical activity was inherently harmful. Studies began to show that regular, moderate exercise could have positive effects on both maternal and fetal health.
- **Guideline Updates:** Health organizations and professional bodies updated their guidelines to reflect new evidence, promoting exercise as a safe and beneficial component of a healthy pregnancy.

The Science Behind Exercise During Pregnancy

Benefits of Exercise

Numerous studies have demonstrated the benefits of exercise during pregnancy:

- **Improved Physical Health:** Regular exercise helps maintain cardiovascular fitness, muscle strength, and flexibility. It can reduce common pregnancy discomforts such as back pain and fatigue.
- **Weight Management:** Exercise supports healthy weight gain during pregnancy. It can help prevent excessive weight gain, which is associated with complications like gestational diabetes and hypertension.
- **Enhanced Mental Well-Being:** Physical activity is known to reduce symptoms of anxiety and depression. Exercise can improve mood, increase energy levels, and promote overall emotional well-being.
- **Reduced Risk of Complications:** Engaging in regular exer-

cise is associated with a lower risk of developing pregnancy-related complications such as preeclampsia and gestational diabetes. It can also help prepare the body for labor and delivery.

Safety Considerations

While exercise is generally safe and beneficial during pregnancy, it is important to consider certain safety guidelines:

- **Consulting Healthcare Providers:** Before starting or continuing an exercise routine, it is advisable for pregnant women to consult their healthcare provider, especially if they have any pre-existing conditions or complications.
- **Avoiding High-Risk Activities:** Certain activities, such as those with a high risk of falling or abdominal trauma, should be avoided. Examples include high-contact sports or activities with a risk of injury.
- **Listening to the Body:** It is important for pregnant women to listen to their bodies and modify or stop exercises if they experience any discomfort, pain, or unusual symptoms.

Guidelines for Safe Exercise During Pregnancy

Types of Safe Exercises

Several types of exercise are recommended for pregnant women due to their low risk and high benefits:

- **Walking:** A low-impact, easily accessible exercise that can be done throughout pregnancy. Walking improves cardiovascular health and can be adapted to individual fitness levels.

- **Swimming:** Provides a full-body workout with minimal impact on the joints. The buoyancy of water supports the body and reduces strain on the back and pelvis.
- **Prenatal Yoga:** Offers gentle stretching, relaxation, and breathing techniques. Prenatal yoga can help with flexibility, balance, and stress relief.
- **Strength Training:** Using light weights or resistance bands to maintain muscle strength. It is important to use proper form and avoid heavy lifting.

Exercise Intensity and Duration

Guidelines suggest aiming for moderate-intensity exercise for at least 150 minutes per week:

- **Moderate Intensity:** Exercise should be done at a pace that allows for conversation but still feels somewhat challenging. Activities should elevate the heart rate without causing excessive fatigue.
- **Duration and Frequency:** Aim for 30 minutes of exercise on most days of the week. It can be broken down into shorter sessions if needed.

Adapting Exercise as Pregnancy Progresses

Pregnancy may bring changes that require modifications to the exercise routine:

- **First Trimester:** Women can generally continue their pre-pregnancy exercise routines, with adjustments as needed for comfort and energy levels.
- **Second Trimester:** As the body undergoes changes, exercises may need to be modified to accommodate a growing

belly and changing balance. It is a good time to focus on core stability and pelvic floor exercises.

- **Third Trimester:** Emphasis should be on exercises that are comfortable and safe, avoiding those that require lying on the back or involve high impact. Focus on gentle stretching, breathing exercises, and maintaining flexibility.

Addressing Common Concerns

Misconceptions About Exercise and Pregnancy

Several misconceptions about exercise during pregnancy persist:

- **Misconception:** Exercise can cause miscarriage.
- **Fact:** There is no evidence to suggest that moderate exercise increases the risk of miscarriage. On the contrary, regular exercise is associated with a lower risk of complications.
- **Misconception:** Pregnant women should avoid exercise to prevent premature labor.
- **Fact:** Exercise does not trigger premature labor in healthy pregnancies. It can help with overall fitness and preparation for labor.
- **Misconception:** Exercise is only for women who were active before pregnancy.
- **Fact:** Pregnant women who were not previously active can start exercising safely. It is important to begin with low-impact activities and gradually increase intensity as tolerated.

Consulting Healthcare Providers

Healthcare providers play a crucial role in guiding safe exercise practices:

- **Individualized Advice:** Providers can offer personalized recommendations based on individual health status, fitness level, and any pregnancy-related conditions.
- **Monitoring and Adjustments:** Regular check-ins with healthcare providers help ensure that the exercise routine remains safe and effective throughout pregnancy.

Promoting Awareness and Education

Educating Expectant Mothers

Educating expectant mothers about the benefits and safety of exercise is essential:

- **Educational Resources:** Providing access to reliable information about exercise during pregnancy helps women make informed decisions.
- **Support Programs:** Prenatal exercise classes and programs offer guidance, support, and community for pregnant women interested in staying active.

Encouraging a Healthy Lifestyle

Encouraging a healthy lifestyle that includes regular exercise supports overall well-being:

- **Holistic Approach:** Combine exercise with other healthy practices such as balanced nutrition, adequate hydration, and stress management for optimal pregnancy health.
- **Long-Term Benefits:** Maintaining an active lifestyle during pregnancy sets a positive precedent for postnatal health and

recovery.

Conclusion

The myth that exercise is dangerous during pregnancy has been debunked by modern medical research, which highlights the numerous benefits of physical activity for both mother and baby. Exercise is a safe and effective way to support physical health, manage weight, and improve mental well-being during pregnancy. By following guidelines for safe exercise and consulting healthcare providers, expectant mothers can enjoy the benefits of physical activity while ensuring a healthy and positive pregnancy experience. Education and awareness are key to dispelling misconceptions and promoting a healthy lifestyle for pregnant women.

Myth-Busting: The Facts Behind Common Misconceptions

Pregnancy is a time filled with excitement and anticipation, but it is also a period when many myths and misconceptions can arise. This myth-busting guide aims to clarify some of the most common misconceptions about pregnancy by providing evidence-based facts. By addressing these myths, expectant mothers and their families can make informed decisions and navigate pregnancy with confidence.

Fact 1: Nutritional Needs During Pregnancy

Myth: You need to "eat for two" during pregnancy.

Fact: While it's true that your caloric and nutritional needs increase during pregnancy, the idea that you need to double your food intake is a misconception.

Understanding Nutritional Needs

- **Caloric Intake:** The recommended additional caloric intake during pregnancy is about 300-350 calories per day, depending on the stage of pregnancy and individual factors. This is roughly equivalent to a healthy snack, not an extra meal.
- **Balanced Diet:** Focus on a balanced diet rich in essential nutrients rather than simply increasing caloric intake. Important nutrients include folic acid, iron, calcium, protein, and omega-3 fatty acids.
- **Healthy Choices:** Prioritize nutrient-dense foods like fruits, vegetables, whole grains, lean proteins, and dairy. Avoid excessive consumption of processed foods and sugary snacks.

Key Takeaways

- **Moderation is Key:** Aim for a moderate increase in calories, focusing on quality over quantity.
- **Nutrient Density:** Choose foods that provide essential nutrients to support both maternal and fetal health.

Fact 2: Cravings and Gender Prediction

Myth: Cravings during pregnancy can predict the baby's gender.

Fact: There is no scientific evidence to support the idea that specific cravings indicate the sex of the baby.

Exploring Cravings

- **Hormonal Changes:** Pregnancy cravings are often influenced by hormonal changes and nutritional needs rather than indicating the baby's gender.
- **Cultural Beliefs:** Many cultures have traditions and folklore that associate cravings with gender prediction, but these are based on anecdotal evidence rather than scientific research.
- **Scientific Perspective:** Research has shown no consistent link between specific food cravings and the baby's sex. Cravings are more likely related to individual dietary preferences and body's nutritional requirements.

Key Takeaways

- **Cravings are Normal:** Pregnancy cravings are a common phenomenon and are not reliable indicators of the baby's gender.
- **Focus on Balanced Diet:** Address cravings with healthy choices and balanced nutrition.

Fact 3: Safe Exercise and Its Benefits

Myth: Exercise is dangerous during pregnancy.

Fact: Exercise is generally safe and beneficial for most pregnant women, with proper precautions and modifications.

Benefits of Exercise

- **Physical Health:** Regular exercise helps maintain cardiovascular health, manage weight, and reduce back pain and fatigue.
- **Mental Well-Being:** Exercise can improve mood, reduce stress, and enhance overall mental well-being.
- **Reduced Risk of Complications:** Engaging in regular, moderate exercise is associated with a lower risk of gestational diabetes, preeclampsia, and preterm labor.

Safety Guidelines

- **Consult Healthcare Providers:** Obtain medical clearance if you have any health concerns or pregnancy-related conditions.
- **Choose Safe Activities:** Opt for low-impact exercises like walking, swimming, and prenatal yoga. Avoid high-risk activities.
- **Listen to Your Body:** Modify or stop exercises if you experience discomfort or unusual symptoms.

Key Takeaways

- **Exercise is Beneficial:** Regular, moderate exercise supports physical and mental health during pregnancy.

- **Follow Safety Guidelines:** Consult healthcare providers and choose safe, appropriate activities.

Fact 4: Heartburn and Hair Growth

Myth: Heartburn during pregnancy means the baby will have lots of hair.

Fact: There is no scientific evidence linking heartburn with the amount of hair a baby will have at birth.

Understanding Heartburn

- **Causes:** Heartburn is commonly caused by hormonal changes and the physical pressure of the growing uterus on the stomach, not by the baby's hair.
- **Fetal Hair Development:** The amount of hair a baby is born with is determined by genetic factors, not by maternal symptoms.

Addressing Heartburn

- **Diet and Lifestyle:** Manage heartburn with dietary adjustments, such as avoiding spicy or acidic foods, and maintaining good posture.
- **Medical Advice:** Seek medical guidance if heartburn is severe or persistent.

Key Takeaways

- **No Link Between Heartburn and Hair:** Heartburn is unrelated to fetal hair growth.
- **Manage Symptoms:** Use dietary and lifestyle changes to

manage heartburn during pregnancy.

Fact 5: Air Travel and Pregnancy Safety

Myth: Pregnant women cannot fly.

Fact: Air travel is generally safe for most pregnant women, especially if they have a healthy pregnancy.

Considerations for Air Travel

- **Airline Policies:** Most airlines allow pregnant women to fly up to around 36 weeks for uncomplicated pregnancies. Check with the airline for specific policies.
- **Health Risks:** While flying is generally safe, consider potential risks such as deep vein thrombosis (DVT) and manage them with proper hydration and movement.
- **Consult Healthcare Providers:** Obtain medical clearance if you have any complications or high-risk conditions.

Practical Tips

- **Comfort:** Choose comfortable seating, stay hydrated, and move around during the flight to prevent discomfort and DVT.
- **Emergency Preparedness:** Know emergency procedures and carry essential medical information.

Key Takeaways

- **Flying is Safe:** For most healthy pregnancies, flying poses minimal risk.
- **Follow Guidelines:** Adhere to airline policies, consult

healthcare providers, and take practical steps to ensure a comfortable journey.

Conclusion

Understanding the facts behind common pregnancy myths helps expectant mothers make informed decisions and reduces unnecessary worry. By dispelling misconceptions about nutritional needs, cravings, exercise, heartburn, and air travel, this guide provides a clearer picture of what to expect during pregnancy. Accurate information and evidence-based guidelines support a healthy and confident pregnancy journey.

Cultural and Historical Perspectives on Pregnancy Myths

Pregnancy myths and beliefs have varied widely across cultures and historical periods. These myths often reflect the values, fears, and understandings of different societies regarding pregnancy and childbirth. By examining ancient beliefs and practices, modern cultural influences, and the impact on expecting mothers across cultures, we gain insight into how cultural contexts shape perceptions of pregnancy.

Ancient Beliefs and Practices

Ancient Egyptian Beliefs

- **Mythological Influences:** In ancient Egypt, pregnancy and childbirth were deeply influenced by mythology. Deities like Tawaret, the goddess of fertility and childbirth, were revered. Pregnant women often invoked her protection to ensure a safe delivery.
  - **Protective Amulets:** Women wore amulets and charms to protect themselves and their babies from evil spirits and potential complications. These items were believed to have magical properties that could influence the health of both mother and child.

Ancient Greek and Roman Practices

- **Divine Intervention:** Ancient Greeks and Romans believed that divine forces played a significant role in pregnancy. For example, they thought that the goddess Artemis could influence childbirth, and prayers or sacrifices were made to gain her favor.

- **Customs and Superstitions:** Various customs and superstitions were observed, such as avoiding certain foods or activities believed to cause harm. The Greeks also practiced a form of prenatal care that included dietary recommendations and specific rituals to ensure a healthy pregnancy.

Medieval European Beliefs

- **Influence of Religion:** During the medieval period, Christian beliefs heavily influenced views on pregnancy. Saints and religious figures were invoked for protection and safe childbirth. Some medieval texts contain detailed advice on managing pregnancy based on religious teachings.
- **Folk Remedies:** Pregnant women often relied on folk remedies and traditional medicine, which included herbal treatments and rituals designed to address common pregnancy symptoms and concerns.

Modern Cultural Influences

Popular Media and Societal Trends

- **Media Representation:** Modern media plays a significant role in shaping cultural perceptions of pregnancy. Television shows, movies, and advertisements often portray pregnancy in ways that can reinforce or challenge existing myths.
- **Celebrity Influence:** Celebrities and public figures can influence pregnancy trends and beliefs through their publicized experiences and endorsements of certain practices or products.

Globalization and Cross-Cultural Exchange

- **Cultural Fusion:** The exchange of cultural practices and beliefs due to globalization has led to a blending of traditional and modern approaches to pregnancy. For example, some cultures incorporate Western prenatal practices while maintaining traditional rituals.
- **Health and Wellness Trends:** The rise of health and wellness trends has brought increased attention to evidence-based practices in pregnancy, sometimes challenging traditional myths and practices.

Technological Advances

- **Medical Technology:** Advances in medical technology, such as ultrasound and genetic testing, have provided more accurate information about pregnancy and fetal development, often debunking traditional myths.
- **Access to Information:** The internet and social media have made information about pregnancy more accessible, allowing for greater dissemination of evidence-based practices and reduction of misinformation.

Impact on Expecting Mothers Across Cultures

Psychological Impact

- **Fear and Anxiety:** Myths and misconceptions about pregnancy can contribute to fear and anxiety among expecting mothers. For example, beliefs about adverse effects of certain activities or foods may lead to unnecessary stress.

- **Cultural Pressure:** Cultural expectations and pressures can influence a mother's experience of pregnancy. In some cultures, there may be strong expectations to adhere to traditional practices or rituals, which can impact a mother's mental and emotional well-being.

Social and Support Systems

- **Community Support:** In many cultures, traditional practices and beliefs are supported by community and family networks. These support systems can provide comfort and reassurance, even if they are based on outdated or incorrect information.
- **Healthcare Access:** The availability and quality of healthcare can vary significantly across cultures. In some areas, traditional practices may supplement or replace modern medical care, influencing the overall experience of pregnancy.

Educational and Informational Gaps

- **Access to Accurate Information:** In cultures with limited access to modern medical information, myths and misconceptions may persist, affecting the quality of prenatal care and maternal health.
- **Education Initiatives:** Efforts to educate expecting mothers about evidence-based practices can help address misconceptions and improve outcomes. Programs that respect cultural beliefs while providing accurate information can be particularly effective.

Conclusion

Cultural and historical perspectives on pregnancy myths reveal a rich tapestry of beliefs and practices that have evolved over time. Ancient practices were influenced by mythology and religion, while modern cultural influences are shaped by media, globalization, and technological advances. Understanding these perspectives helps us appreciate the diverse ways in which cultures view pregnancy and the impact of myths on expecting mothers. By bridging the gap between traditional beliefs and evidence-based practices, we can support a more informed and positive pregnancy experience for women around the world.

The Science Behind Pregnancy Facts

Understanding the scientific basis behind pregnancy facts is crucial for ensuring a healthy and informed pregnancy. This section delves into the role of nutrition and dietary guidelines, exercise recommendations and research, and the impact of hormonal changes on physical symptoms.

The Role of Nutrition and Dietary Guidelines

Nutritional Needs During Pregnancy

- **Increased Caloric Intake:** During pregnancy, the body requires additional calories to support fetal growth and maternal health. The general recommendation is an increase of about 300-350 calories per day in the second and third trimesters. However, this does not mean doubling food intake; rather, it involves focusing on nutrient-dense foods.
- **Essential Nutrients:**
- **Folic Acid:** Critical for preventing neural tube defects, folic acid should be consumed in higher amounts (about 600-

800 micrograms daily) through supplements and foods like leafy greens, fortified cereals, and legumes.

- **Iron:** Increased blood volume during pregnancy demands more iron. The recommended intake is around 27 milligrams per day, with sources including red meat, poultry, fish, and fortified cereals.
- **Calcium:** Essential for the development of the baby's bones and teeth, the recommended calcium intake is about 1,000 milligrams daily, provided through dairy products, fortified plant-based milks, and leafy greens.
- **Protein:** Necessary for fetal growth and tissue development, pregnant women should aim for about 71 grams of protein daily from sources like lean meats, beans, nuts, and eggs.
- **Omega-3 Fatty Acids:** Important for fetal brain development, omega-3s can be found in fatty fish, flaxseeds, and walnuts.

Dietary Guidelines

- **Balanced Diet:** Emphasize a diet rich in fruits, vegetables, whole grains, lean proteins, and healthy fats. A well-rounded diet helps meet increased nutritional needs and supports overall health.
- **Hydration:** Staying well-hydrated is crucial. Pregnant women should aim to drink at least 8-10 cups of fluids daily, with water being the best option.
- **Avoiding Harmful Substances:** Limit caffeine intake to about 200 milligrams per day, avoid alcohol, and stay away from high-risk foods like raw seafood and undercooked meats to reduce the risk of foodborne illnesses.

Exercise Recommendations and Research

Benefits of Exercise During Pregnancy

- **Physical Health:** Regular exercise helps manage weight, improves cardiovascular health, and reduces the risk of gestational diabetes and preeclampsia. It also alleviates common discomforts such as back pain and fatigue.
- **Mental Well-Being:** Exercise has been shown to reduce symptoms of anxiety and depression, improve mood, and enhance overall mental well-being.
- **Labor and Delivery:** Regular physical activity can improve endurance and strength, potentially leading to a smoother labor process. It may also reduce the likelihood of cesarean delivery and shorten recovery time postpartum.

Safe Exercise Guidelines

- **Types of Exercise:** Low-impact activities such as walking, swimming, and prenatal yoga are generally recommended. These activities provide cardiovascular benefits and improve flexibility and strength without excessive strain.
- **Intensity and Duration:** Aim for at least 150 minutes of moderate-intensity exercise per week, as recommended by the American College of Obstetricians and Gynecologists (ACOG). Adjust intensity based on comfort and fitness level.
- **Safety Precautions:** Avoid activities with a high risk of falling or injury, such as contact sports or high-intensity interval training. Ensure proper hydration and listen to your body, modifying or stopping exercises if any discomfort arises.

Research Findings

- **Gestational Diabetes:** Studies show that regular exercise can help manage blood sugar levels and reduce the risk of gestational diabetes.
- **Preterm Birth:** Some research suggests that exercise may lower the risk of preterm birth by promoting overall health and reducing stress.
- **Mental Health:** Exercise is associated with lower levels of prenatal depression and anxiety, supporting emotional health during pregnancy.

Hormonal Changes and Physical Symptoms

Hormonal Changes During Pregnancy

- **Estrogen and Progesterone:** These hormones play crucial roles in maintaining pregnancy. Estrogen supports uterine growth and fetal development, while progesterone helps relax the uterine muscles and supports implantation.
- **Human Chorionic Gonadotropin (hCG):** Produced by the placenta, hCG is essential for maintaining progesterone levels and is used as an indicator in pregnancy tests.
- **Relaxin:** This hormone helps relax the ligaments and joints in preparation for childbirth and can contribute to physical symptoms such as pelvic pain.

Common Physical Symptoms

- **Nausea and Vomiting:** Often referred to as morning sickness, nausea and vomiting are common in the first trimester due to hormonal changes. This condition usually subsides after the first trimester for most women.

- **Heartburn:** Caused by the relaxation of the lower esophageal sphincter due to increased progesterone levels and physical pressure from the growing uterus, heartburn is a common symptom in the later stages of pregnancy.
- **Fatigue:** Increased progesterone levels and the body's efforts to support the growing fetus can lead to significant fatigue, particularly in the first and third trimesters.
- **Swelling:** Hormonal changes and increased blood volume can cause swelling in the legs and feet. This condition, known as edema, is usually more pronounced in the later stages of pregnancy.
- **Back Pain:** The growing uterus and hormonal changes can affect the alignment of the spine and pelvis, leading to back pain. Strengthening core muscles and practicing good posture can help alleviate discomfort.

Conclusion

Understanding the science behind pregnancy facts is essential for making informed decisions and ensuring a healthy pregnancy. Nutrition plays a critical role in supporting both maternal and fetal health, while exercise offers numerous benefits when performed safely. Hormonal changes significantly impact physical symptoms, and awareness of these changes can help manage common discomforts. By focusing on evidence-based practices and guidelines, expectant mothers can navigate pregnancy with confidence and promote their well-being and that of their baby.

Expert Opinions and Medical Advice

Pregnancy involves various physical, emotional, and lifestyle changes, making expert guidance crucial for expectant mothers. In this section, we explore expert opinions and medical advice from obstetricians and gynecologists, insights from nutritionists and fitness experts, and real-life experiences from expecting mothers to provide a comprehensive view of pregnancy management.

Interviews with Obstetricians and Gynecologists

Common Concerns Addressed

1. **Prenatal Care and Routine Screenings:**

• **Dr. Emily Johnson, OB-GYN:** "Routine prenatal care is essential for monitoring both maternal and fetal health. Regular check-ups help identify potential issues early and allow for timely interventions. Standard screenings include blood tests, ultrasounds, and gestational diabetes testing, which are crucial for ensuring a healthy pregnancy."

1. **Managing Pregnancy Symptoms:**

• **Dr. Robert Smith, OB-GYN:** "Common pregnancy symptoms like nausea, fatigue, and back pain are often manageable with lifestyle adjustments and medical advice. For severe symptoms, we explore options such as medication or physical therapy. It's important for pregnant women to communicate openly about their symptoms to receive appropriate care."

1. **Exercise and Activity Recommendations:**

· **Dr. Laura Kim, OB-GYN:** "Exercise is generally safe and beneficial for most pregnant women. We recommend moderate-intensity activities like walking and swimming. However, each pregnancy is unique, and women with complications or high-risk factors should seek personalized advice before starting or continuing an exercise routine."

1. **Travel During Pregnancy:**

· **Dr. Michael Lee, OB-GYN:** "Flying during pregnancy is safe for most women, especially if they are healthy and have no complications. We advise taking precautions to prevent deep vein thrombosis and ensuring comfort during the flight. Pregnant women should also be aware of airline policies and consult their healthcare provider if traveling close to their due date."

Insights from Nutritionists and Fitness Experts

Nutrition During Pregnancy

1. **Dietary Guidelines and Essential Nutrients:**

· **Registered Dietitian Sarah Williams:** "A well-balanced diet is critical during pregnancy. Focus on consuming a variety of nutrient-dense foods, including fruits, vegetables, lean proteins, and whole grains. Key nutrients like folic acid, iron, calcium, and omega-3 fatty acids support fetal development and maternal health."

1. **Managing Cravings and Dietary Restrictions:**

· **Nutritionist Rebecca Patel:** "Cravings are common, but it's important to make healthy choices. If a craving leads to an unhealthy food choice, try to balance it with nutritious options throughout the day. For women with dietary restrictions or specific health conditions, tailored nutritional plans can help meet their needs while maintaining a healthy pregnancy."

1. **Hydration and Fluid Intake:**

· **Nutritionist James Turner:** "Adequate hydration is crucial. Pregnant women should aim for at least 8-10 cups of fluids daily. Water is the best choice, but other fluids like herbal teas and milk also contribute to overall hydration. Proper fluid intake supports amniotic fluid levels and helps prevent common issues like constipation."

Exercise Recommendations

1. **Safe Exercise Practices:**

· **Fitness Expert Amanda Brooks:** "Pregnant women should engage in low-impact activities that they enjoy and are comfortable with. Activities like walking, swimming, and prenatal yoga are excellent choices. It's important to listen to your body, avoid high-risk activities, and adjust intensity as needed."

1. **Benefits of Regular Physical Activity:**

- **Fitness Trainer Michael Davis:** "Regular exercise during pregnancy offers numerous benefits, including improved cardiovascular health, reduced risk of gestational diabetes, and enhanced mood. It also helps prepare the body for labor and delivery. Consistency and moderation are key to achieving these benefits."

Real-Life Experiences from Expecting Mothers

Personal Stories and Insights

1. **Managing Pregnancy Symptoms:**

- **Emily Thompson, Expecting Mother:** "I experienced severe morning sickness during my first trimester. I found that eating small, frequent meals and staying hydrated helped manage the nausea. My OB-GYN also recommended some over-the-counter remedies, which provided relief."

1. **Balancing Exercise and Rest:**

- **Sophie Green, Expecting Mother:** "Staying active was important to me, but I also had to learn to listen to my body. I enjoyed prenatal yoga, which helped with flexibility and relaxation. On days when I felt particularly tired, I allowed myself to rest and adjusted my routine accordingly."

1. **Diet and Nutrition Challenges:**

- **Rachel Adams, Expecting Mother:** "Cravings were a big challenge for me, especially for sweets. I tried to satisfy my cravings with healthier alternatives like fruit or yogurt. My nutritionist helped me create a meal plan that balanced indulgences with nutrient-rich foods."

1. **Travel Experience:**

- **Ava Martinez, Expecting Mother:** "I traveled by plane during my second trimester and found it to be manageable. I made sure to stay hydrated, walked around the cabin periodically, and followed my doctor's advice on travel. It was a great experience overall, and I felt well-prepared."

Conclusion

Expert opinions and medical advice from obstetricians, gynecologists, nutritionists, and fitness experts provide valuable insights into managing pregnancy. From routine prenatal care and symptom management to dietary guidelines and safe exercise practices, these perspectives help expectant mothers navigate their pregnancy with informed confidence. Real-life experiences further illustrate how individuals adapt to the challenges and joys of pregnancy, offering practical advice and support for others on the same journey. By integrating expert guidance and personal experiences, expectant mothers can make well-informed decisions that promote a healthy and positive pregnancy experience.

Practical Tips for Navigating Pregnancy Information

N avigating pregnancy information can be overwhelm-ing due to the abundance of advice, myths, and recommendations available. To ensure you are making informed decisions, it is essential to distinguish between fact and fiction, utilize reliable sources, and effectively address concerns with your healthcare provider. Here are some practical tips to help you manage pregnancy information effectively.

How to Distinguish Between Fact and Fiction

1. Evaluate the Source

- **Credibility:** Consider the credibility of the source providing the information. Trusted sources include medical institu-tions, government health agencies (like the CDC or WHO), and accredited health organizations. Avoid relying on anecdotal evidence or information from unverified websites or social media.

- **Expert Opinions:** Look for information authored or reviewed by medical professionals such as obstetricians, gynecologists, or registered dietitians. Expert opinions are based on scientific research and clinical experience.

2. Check for Evidence-Based Information

- **Scientific Research:** Reliable pregnancy information is typically supported by scientific research and clinical studies. Check if the information references peer-reviewed studies or clinical trials.
- **Consistent Recommendations:** Verify if the advice is consistent with current guidelines from reputable health organizations like the American College of Obstetricians and Gynecologists (ACOG) or the National Institutes of Health (NIH).

3. Beware of Common Myths

- **Myth vs. Fact:** Be cautious of common myths and misconceptions that circulate widely. Myths often lack scientific backing and can lead to unnecessary worry or misinformation.
- **Critical Thinking:** Use critical thinking to assess the validity of pregnancy-related claims. If something sounds too good to be true or contradicts established medical guidelines, it's worth further investigation.

4. Consult Reliable Books and Resources

- **Books by Experts:** Books written by healthcare professionals or academic experts can provide reliable information. Ensure that the authors are recognized in their field and that the book is up-to-date.

- **Educational Websites:** Websites from reputable health organizations or educational institutions often offer accurate and current information. Look for sections specifically dedicated to pregnancy and prenatal care.

Reliable Sources for Pregnancy Information

1. **Medical Institutions and Government Health Agencies**

- **Centers for Disease Control and Prevention (CDC):** Offers comprehensive information on pregnancy health, including guidelines, vaccines, and health tips.
- **World Health Organization (WHO):** Provides global health guidelines and recommendations on pregnancy and maternal health.
- **National Institutes of Health (NIH):** Offers detailed resources and research findings on pregnancy-related topics.

2. **Professional Medical Associations**

- **American College of Obstetricians and Gynecologists (ACOG):** Provides evidence-based guidelines, patient education materials, and expert advice on various aspects of pregnancy and childbirth.
- **Academy of Nutrition and Dietetics:** Offers nutrition-related information and resources specifically tailored for pregnant women.
- **American Pregnancy Association:** Provides educational

resources, articles, and FAQs on pregnancy-related topics.

3. **Healthcare Providers**

- **Obstetricians and Gynecologists:** Your primary healthcare provider is an invaluable resource for personalized advice and information tailored to your specific situation.
- **Registered Dietitians:** For dietary concerns and nutritional advice, consulting a registered dietitian with experience in prenatal nutrition can be highly beneficial.
- **Certified Fitness Trainers:** For exercise recommendations and safety during pregnancy, seek advice from fitness trainers who specialize in prenatal fitness.

Addressing Concerns with Your Healthcare Provider

1. **Prepare for Your Appointments**

- **List Your Questions:** Before your appointment, make a list of questions or concerns you have about your pregnancy. This ensures that you address all your issues and do not forget important topics during the visit.
- **Record Symptoms:** Keep a record of any symptoms or changes you experience. This can help your healthcare provider diagnose and address any issues more effectively.

2. **Communicate Openly**

- **Be Honest:** Share all relevant information about your health, lifestyle, and any symptoms you are experiencing. Honesty allows your provider to give you the most accurate and tailored advice.

- **Discuss Concerns:** If you have doubts about any recommendations or information, discuss them openly with your healthcare provider. They can provide clarification and reassurance.

3. Seek Second Opinions if Needed

- **Different Perspectives:** If you are unsure about a diagnosis or treatment plan, seeking a second opinion can provide additional perspectives and help you make a more informed decision.
- **Specialist Consultations:** For complex issues or specific concerns, consider consulting specialists such as maternal-fetal medicine experts or nutritionists.

4. Understand Your Options

- **Informed Decisions:** Ensure that you understand all your options regarding prenatal care, testing, and interventions. Ask about the benefits, risks, and alternatives to make well-informed decisions.
- **Clarify Procedures:** If your healthcare provider recommends specific procedures or tests, ask for detailed explanations about why they are necessary and what to expect.

Conclusion

Navigating pregnancy information requires careful evaluation of sources, reliance on evidence-based practices, and open communication with healthcare providers. By distinguishing between fact and fiction, using reliable sources, and addressing concerns effectively, expectant mothers can make informed decisions that support their health and well-being. Accurate information and proactive engagement with healthcare professionals ensure a positive and well-managed pregnancy experience.

Case Studies and Personal Stories

Exploring personal experiences and case studies can provide valuable insights into how women navigate and overcome pregnancy myths. By examining stories of women who have debunked common myths and lessons learned from their journeys, we can gain a deeper understanding of the impact of these myths on real-life experiences.

Experiences of Women Who Debunked Myths

Case Study 1: Debunking the "You're Eating for Two" Myth

Background: Sarah, a 32-year-old expecting mother, was initially overwhelmed by the idea that she needed to consume double the amount of food to support her pregnancy. This myth led her to overeat and gain excessive weight during her first trimester.

Experience:

- **Initial Belief:** Sarah believed that eating twice as much was necessary for her and her baby's health. She often indulged in high-calorie foods and snacks.

- **Realization:** After gaining more weight than recommended and experiencing discomfort, Sarah sought advice from a registered dietitian.
- **Outcome:** The dietitian clarified that while caloric needs increase, they only slightly, and emphasized the importance of a balanced diet with nutrient-dense foods rather than excessive calories. Sarah adjusted her eating habits, focusing on portion control and healthier choices.

Lesson Learned: Sarah's experience highlights the importance of understanding that while nutritional needs do increase during pregnancy, it is not about doubling food intake but rather making healthier, balanced choices.

Case Study 2: Overcoming the "Cravings Predict Baby's Gender" Myth

Background: Maria, a 28-year-old first-time mother, was convinced that her strong cravings for sweet foods meant she was having a girl, based on an old wives' tale she heard.

Experience:

- **Initial Belief:** Maria had strong cravings for sweets and was excited to learn whether this predicted the gender of her baby.
- **Realization:** Despite her cravings, Maria's ultrasound revealed that she was expecting a boy. She realized that cravings have no scientific basis in predicting a baby's gender.
- **Outcome:** Maria learned to enjoy her cravings in moderation and focused on evidence-based methods for understanding her pregnancy and preparing for childbirth.

Lesson Learned: This story underscores the importance of distinguishing between folklore and scientifically validated information. Cravings are normal but do not indicate the baby's gender.

Case Study 3: Navigating the "Exercise is Dangerous During Pregnancy" Myth

Background: Jessica, a 35-year-old fitness enthusiast, was concerned about continuing her exercise routine when she became pregnant due to widespread beliefs that exercise could harm the baby.

Experience:

- **Initial Belief:** Jessica considered halting her fitness routine entirely out of fear that it might negatively impact her pregnancy.
- **Realization:** After consulting with her obstetrician and a prenatal fitness trainer, Jessica learned that moderate exercise was not only safe but beneficial. She was advised on how to adapt her workouts to suit her changing body.
- **Outcome:** Jessica continued her exercise routine with modifications and found that it helped her manage stress, maintain energy levels, and prepare for labor.

Lesson Learned: Jessica's experience demonstrates that exercise, when done correctly and under professional guidance, is generally safe and beneficial during pregnancy, contrary to the myth that it is dangerous.

Case Study 4: Challenging the "Heartburn Means Your Baby Will Have Lots of Hair" Myth

Background: Emily, a 30-year-old expecting mother, was told that her frequent heartburn indicated she would have a baby with a full head of hair, a popular myth she heard from friends and family.

Experience:

- **Initial Belief:** Emily was curious and somewhat anxious about the accuracy of the myth. She experienced significant heartburn throughout her pregnancy.
- **Realization:** After her baby was born, she found that the amount of hair was not linked to her heartburn at all. Her healthcare provider explained that heartburn is more commonly related to hormonal changes and pressure from the growing uterus.
- **Outcome:** Emily's experience led her to understand that such myths are not based on scientific evidence and to focus on managing heartburn through recommended dietary and lifestyle changes.

Lesson Learned: Emily's story highlights how common pregnancy myths can lead to unnecessary concern and emphasizes the importance of relying on medical advice for managing pregnancy symptoms.

Case Study 5: Clarifying the "You Can't Fly While Pregnant" Myth

Background: Laura, a 29-year-old professional, was advised by some friends and family that air travel was unsafe during pregnancy, causing her to worry about her planned business trip.

Experience:

- **Initial Belief:** Laura initially avoided booking flights for work trips, fearing potential risks associated with air travel during pregnancy.

- **Realization:** After consulting her healthcare provider, Laura learned that air travel is generally safe for most pregnant women, especially if they are healthy and follow certain precautions.
- **Outcome:** Laura traveled during her second trimester, following advice to stay hydrated, move around periodically, and wear compression stockings. The trip went smoothly, and she felt reassured by the evidence-based guidance.

Lesson Learned: Laura's experience illustrates that while travel during pregnancy is often safe, it's important to consult with healthcare providers and follow specific precautions rather than relying on general myths or advice.

Lessons Learned from Personal Journeys

1. **Importance of Evidence-Based Information:** Many personal stories reveal that myths and misconceptions can lead to unnecessary anxiety or incorrect practices. Relying on evidence-based information and expert advice helps make informed decisions and reduces stress.
2. **Communication with Healthcare Providers:** Open communication with healthcare providers is crucial for understanding and managing pregnancy-related concerns. Personal experiences demonstrate the value of discussing symptoms, fears, and myths with professionals who can offer personalized guidance.
3. **Adaptation and Flexibility:** Pregnancy is a time of change, and being open to adapting routines and expectations based on accurate information can lead to a healthier and

more positive experience. Personal stories often highlight the benefits of flexibility and the importance of adjusting to new insights.

4. **Self-Education and Critical Thinking:** Women who actively seek out reliable information and question myths often feel more empowered and prepared. Personal experiences underscore the role of self-education and critical thinking in navigating pregnancy.

Conclusion

Case studies and personal stories provide valuable perspectives on how pregnancy myths can impact experiences and decisions. By exploring these narratives, we gain insights into the importance of relying on accurate information, consulting healthcare professionals, and remaining adaptable. Personal journeys offer practical lessons that can help others make informed choices and enjoy a healthier, more positive pregnancy experience.

Conclusion

Navigating pregnancy involves a mix of anticipation, excitement, and uncertainty, influenced by a plethora of information and myths. Understanding the truth behind common misconceptions, relying on credible sources, and seeking expert advice are essential for ensuring a healthy and informed pregnancy journey.

Key Takeaways

1. **Distinguishing Fact from Fiction:** Pregnancy myths often circulate due to cultural traditions or anecdotal experiences. It's crucial to differentiate between these myths and scientifically validated information. Evaluating the credibility of sources and understanding the basis of advice helps in making informed decisions.

2. **Utilizing Reliable Sources:** Trusted resources, including medical institutions, professional associations, and healthcare providers, offer accurate and evidence-based information. Relying on these sources ensures that the advice and guidance you follow are rooted in scientific research and clinical expertise.

3. **Addressing Concerns with Healthcare Providers:** Open communication with obstetricians, gynecologists, nutritionists, and fitness experts is vital. Discussing any concerns or questions with healthcare providers allows for personalized advice tailored to your specific needs and circumstances.

4. **Learning from Personal Experiences:** Personal stories and case studies provide real-life insights into how women navigate and overcome pregnancy myths. These experiences highlight the importance of evidence-based practices and

the value of flexibility and self-education.

5. **Practical Strategies:** Implementing practical strategies, such as preparing for appointments, questioning and understanding medical advice, and seeking second opinions, can enhance the pregnancy experience and ensure that you are well-informed and supported.

Final Thoughts

Pregnancy is a transformative and deeply personal journey, and having accurate information is key to navigating it successfully. By debunking myths, relying on trusted sources, and engaging with healthcare professionals, expectant mothers can make empowered decisions that contribute to their well-being and that of their baby. Embracing evidence-based practices and learning from others' experiences fosters a positive and informed approach to pregnancy, leading to a healthier and more fulfilling experience.

In conclusion, staying informed, questioning myths, and seeking expert guidance will help ensure that the journey through pregnancy is as smooth, healthy, and joyful as possible.